Table of contents

Quotation

"The darkest thing about Africa has always been our ignorance of it."

George Kimble b. 1912

MAP OF AFRICA

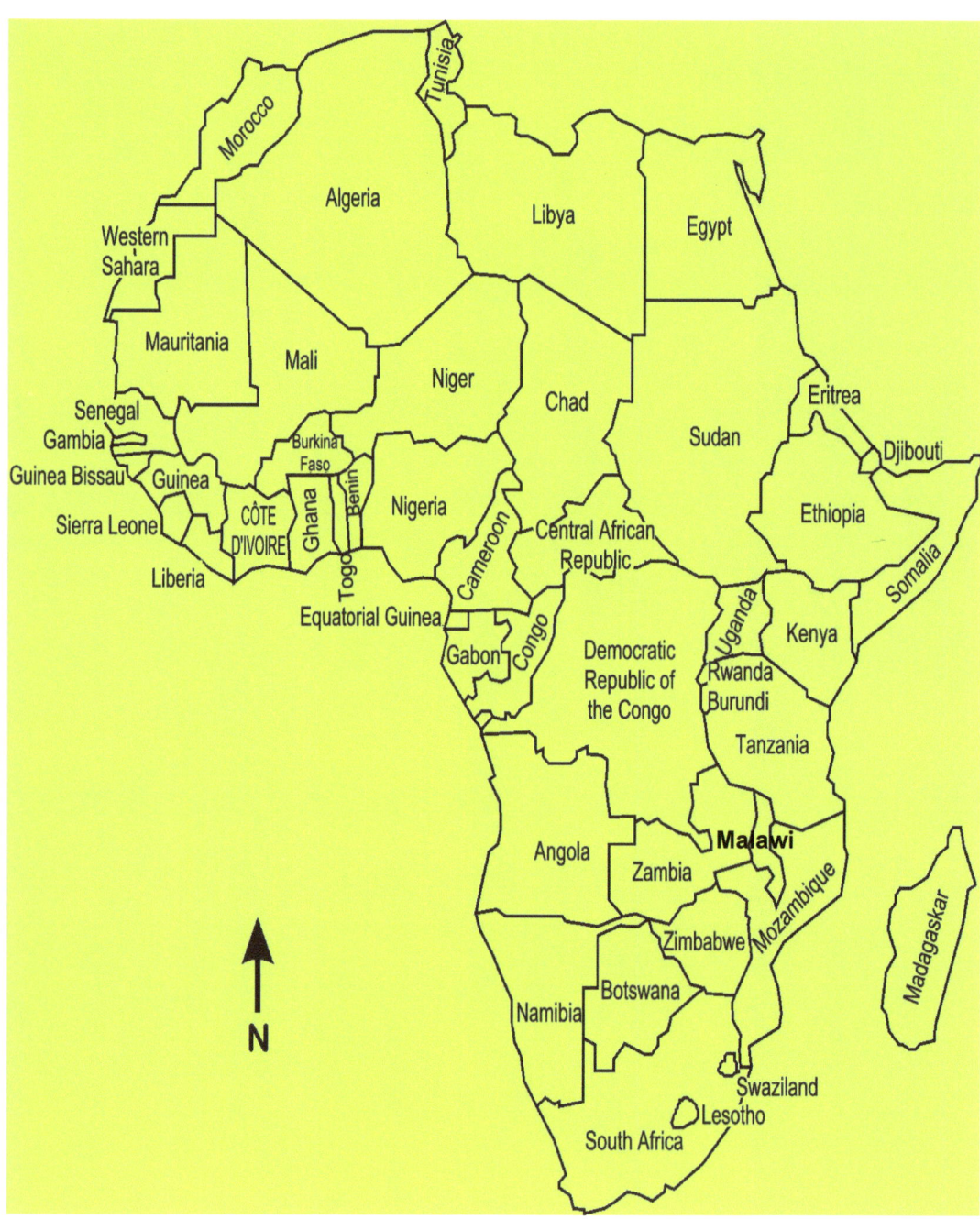

Cnx.org

Foreword

There is limited information on African cultural traditions and its influence on pregnancy in the United Kingdom. It is acknowledged that cultural knowledge is significant in healthcare provision. In recent times it has become more relevant due to the diverse ethnic population that has migrated into the United Kingdom over the last few decades; however Africa is a vast continent with many different languages, traditions and cultures. To engage with black African women effectively, particularly newly arrived immigrants, some knowledge of their culture is required. It would be beneficial to differentiate between particular countries and realise the relevance of certain cultural norms.

General African knowledge is important; it encompasses popular cultural norms such as dress and diet. However, culture specific knowledge of Africa addresses certain taboos and restrictions that are adhered too and which may affect individuals' health choices. This book contains culture- specific and generic knowledge on black African culture specific to pregnancy. It is hoped that this knowledge will facilitate health professionals in meeting the healthcare needs of black African women in a holistic manner.

Introduction

The root of the matter

Health professionals on a daily basis deal with different cultures and its complexities and these problems should always be tackled with critical awareness. A health professional should be sensitive to the socio-cultural context of women when providing care and be aware of the power struggles that women may face. Health professionals can utilise cultural knowledge to eliminate health disparities, facilitate informed choice and offer support to black African women during pregnancy. Appropriate advice and choice cannot be offered to these women if information given is not culturally sensitive. Provision of maternity services, which are culturally sensitive, will improve contact between these vulnerable women and all health professionals.

Section One

1.1 Africa - the root of the culture

Africa is the second largest and most populated continent in the world. The cultures and peoples of Africa are varied and diverse. The various cultures of Africa have many similarities, yet there are subtle differences. A non-native may assume that all African countries have the same culture, but after further exploration the culture in different countries may be seen as being vastly different.

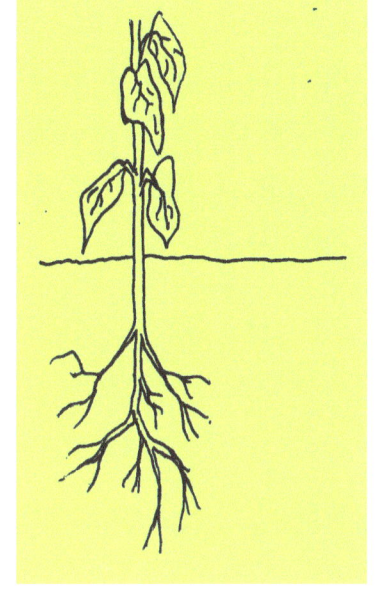

cnx.org

Culture is displayed in many layers and levels one may use the analogy of a plant to describe the different layers of culture. The seed of the plant is the primary level of culture, it contains the information that forms a culture. This information is hidden and it is difficult to determine what nature of plant will develop from the seed. This seed contains all the cultural practices and traditions that have been passed down from generation to generation. This information is privy only those who are born into the culture. This hidden culture is private and secret and rarely spoken about to outsiders.

The roots that materialises from the seed may begin to illustrate to the outsider the nature of the plant, however identifying the plant is concealed until tendrils begin to emerge above ground level. This may be compared to culture whereby some parts are exposed to outsiders due to the fact that they are visible. For instance, individuals from some cultures perform common rituals that are continued although they have become westernised or are living in foreign societies. These rituals may be the observance of cultural festivals and celebrations.

The plant that will eventually be established from the seed is visible to all and is easily identified. Individuals from particular cultures may be identified if they maintain their traditional dress, eat their traditional foods and listen to their cultural music. An outsider can identify with this variation and see what makes this culture different from others. Hence, the culture may be distinguishable and more easily classed.

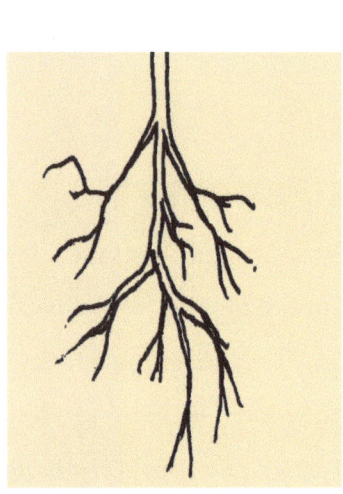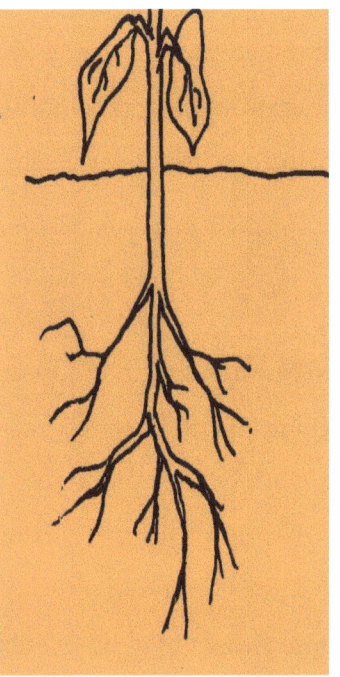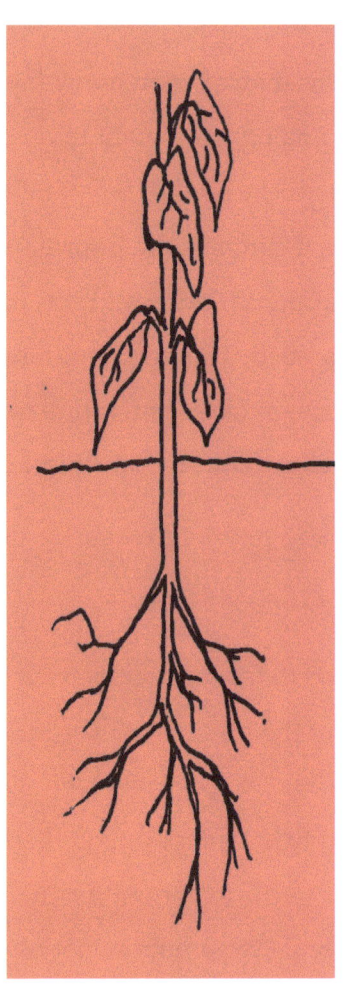

cnx.org

1.2 Africa as a forest of culture

Black Africa can be divided into four parts, West Africa, East Africa, Central Africa and Southern Africa. In each part there are countries that have some similarities in their culture. One reason for this similarity, is that Africa had no definable countries and boundaries until colonisation. During colonisation lines were cut across traditional borders, ignoring ethnic, linguistic and cultural groups mainly for administrative convenience (1). Consequently, cultural groups occupying different countries share similarities in their rituals and practices. This is observed in East Africa, otherwise known as the horn of Africa where Ethiopia, Eritrea and Somalia have similar traits in language, customs and foods.

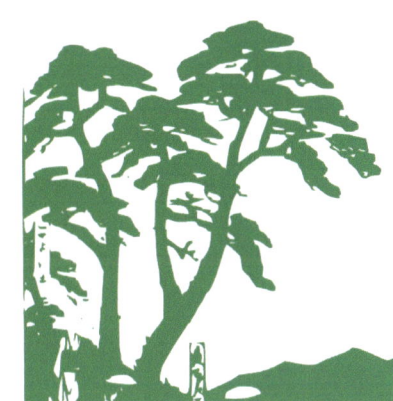

Clker.com

Pre-colonial Africa possessed as many as 10,000 states including small nomadic tribes, the large Bantu-speaking people of central and South Africa and the autonomous Yoruba group of West Africa (1). The transatlantic slave trade was influential in dispersing cultural groups. Warring between different tribal groups often resulted in defeated tribes being enslaved and sold off or traded to other tribes and to Europeans in exchange for merchandise. Many tribes were distributed far from their roots causing the spread of culture and tradition to different parts of Africa.

Decolonisation occurred when western educated African men showed potential for leadership, which allowed countries to take administrative control and become independent of European rule (1). Due to the nineteenth century colonisation of Africa a few European languages are still dominant in Africa. In particular, English and French share official status with native indigenous languages in many countries in Africa. The practice of western religions such as Christianity, mainly bought to Africa by missionaries was previously unknown to most Africans. Prior to colonisation tribal religions and Islam were the main religions, which some Africans have continued to practice to this present day.

Traditional Medicine

Traditional medicine plays an important role in many developing countries. It is estimated that 70% to 80% of Africans make use of traditional medicine (2). Traditional medicine as conceived by the World health Organisation (WHO), is the diagnosis, prevention and elimination of physical and mental imbalance relying exclusively on practical experience and observation passed down from generation to generation whether verbally or in writing (3). Illness is seen by Africans as a supernatural phenomenon governed by a hierarchy of vital powers, beginning with the most powerful deity. Traditional medicine has a base belief of the interaction between the spiritual and physical well-being. Holistic approaches are used in dealing with health and ill health (2). The traditional healing process follows various stages

- Identification of the cause of illness either by divination
- Removal of the cause by neutralization or seeking forgiveness by sacrifice, rituals or prescription of certain medicines.

Traditional medicine is normally practiced by traditional doctors, witch doctors and persons believed to have special powers. These persons are known within communities and access is normally made by self-referral.

There are several factors that may affect an individual's culture in the diaspora, including their experience on contact with the ethnic group in the country of arrival and the ties with the country they have left behind. It is important to note that some cultural practices are still relevant no matter whether an individual resides in Africa or the United Kingdom. Firstly, Africa has a largely paternalistic culture; subsequently men are usually the decision makers in all aspects of family life. Secondly, elders are still greatly respected in African culture and children and marriage are still important aspects for every community.

1.3 The migration of African culture

The migration of African women to the UK appears to be motivated by two major forces, economic and political (4). The majority of these women have migrated during the most economically active period of their lives, which has coincided with their reproductive years. Hence, these women have had to deal with the life changing effects of both migration and childbearing, which could have consequences on their well being.

Many African women commence child bearing at an early age and bear many children in their lifetime (5). There is a greater likelihood of these women having to work as well as continue childbearing. This point is most likely to apply to first generation Africans rather than the second generation Africans (Second generation Africans are individuals born in the UK to migrant African parents). Higher parity is one factor that puts black African women at greater risk of morbidity and mortality; other factors are low economic status and pre existing disease. African women are known to be at greater risk of pregnancy related diseases such as pre eclampsia and gestational diabetes (6). Poorer socio economic and other underlying health problems mean that black African women appear to be in a higher risk category than any other ethnic groups.

Black African women who are new immigrants or asylum seekers also pose several issues to healthcare services. These women constitute a relatively new maternity client group (5). There is little literature that explores their health status prior to their arrival in the UK. It is accepted that African refugee women are particularly vulnerable to poorer health related to poor pre-conceptual care. There may be a range of disorders or conditions that these women present with such as malaria, human immunodeficiency virus, female genital alteration, tuberculosis and anaemia. Newly migrant women may have a lack of knowledge of how the health care service works within the UK. Fear and anxiety may also influence their health seeking behaviour whether due to unfamiliarity of the system or fear of prosecution if seeking asylum. All these factors are the underlying problems, which may prevent these women from approaching heath services for care or advice. If access is made then other issues may arise, these number from language/ communication barriers to culturally insensitive services.

There are more African people living in London than any other part of the UK (7, 8). The biggest groups of Africans living in London are Kenyans, Nigerians, Ugandans and Somalians. There are also smaller pockets of Cameroonians, Ghanaians, Malawians and Zimbabweans. These cultures will be discussed in greater detail looking at influences on health seeking behaviour and common practices in pregnancy and childbirth. Attempts will be made to give some insight into African culture and how this knowledge can help health professionals engage with black African pregnant women.

1.4 Culturally competent care

To deliver culturally competent care, health professionals do not necessarily have to have expert knowledge of all cultures. If there is regular contact within the health care setting with specific groups of women then some knowledge of their common cultural practices is beneficial. In order to ensure that care is culturally sensitive the woman's needs and expectations need to be met as far as possible. It is unreasonable for black African women to expect the UK health care system to cater to all their cultural needs. However, there should be respect, compromise and acknowledgement from healthcare professionals of these cultural needs. Cultural knowledge should be used as a springboard in order to overcome any misconceptions (9).

Asking questions about a woman's culture will demonstrate a health professional's interest and will facilitate greater understanding of the woman's needs. Questions may be specific or general depending on the circumstances. Listed below are some examples of questions, which may be beneficial for a midwife to ask women.

1. What foods do you commonly eat whilst pregnant?
2. Who do you expect will provide medical care?
3. Is the gender of the health professional important to you?
4. Are you able to keep your appointments, do you know why they are important?
5. After birth are there any special rituals that has to be performed for the baby?
6. In your culture do you give baby colostrum?
7. Who cares for the mother after birth?
9. Is it okay to praise the baby after birth (9)

1.5 Barriers to healthcare

Culture is one of several barriers which woman face when trying to access healthcare services. Healthcare professionals can also create barriers to woman accessing healthcare services. The following scenarios may highlight some of these barriers:

Scenario one

Tunde a 30-year-old Nigerian woman has newly arrived in the UK and is currently 10 weeks pregnant. She is aware that she needs to see someone for antenatal care. However, in her country this may not be done until the second trimester. Tunde is unaware that she is needs to register with a GP and has decided that if there any concerns about the pregnancy she will go to the hospital. In the meanwhile there is no need to seek any healthcare. Her main priority now is to get used to living in the UK.

Scenario two

A Somali woman named Farah is having her fourth child and has already been to her GP to arrange referral to her local hospital. There was a delay with the GP in sending her referral letter. She has been posted a booking appointment for four weeks time when she is 16 weeks. Farah and her husband do not speak English very well and when she arrives for her booking appointment, an interpreter has not been arranged. The GP had failed to notify the hospital that Farah and her husband do not speak good English. Subsequently, the appointment has to be rearranged for when she is 19 weeks nearly half way through her pregnancy.

The next two pages display the cultural and health professional barriers that may be present when accessing health care.

In the two scenarios which examples of barriers may be present? What methods can be used to reduce or remove these barriers?

Cultural barriers to maternity services

Maternity Services

BARRIERS

Belief in fate

Women's issues

Fears about maternity care

Privacy

Dependence on community

Pregnancy is a normal process not requiring any monitoring

Fear of caesarean Birth

Arranging a chaperone

Contact with men other than husband

Immigration fears

Family gatekeepers

Adapted from MEDACT, Access to Maternity Services, Barriers created by culture 2009

Barriers created by health professionals

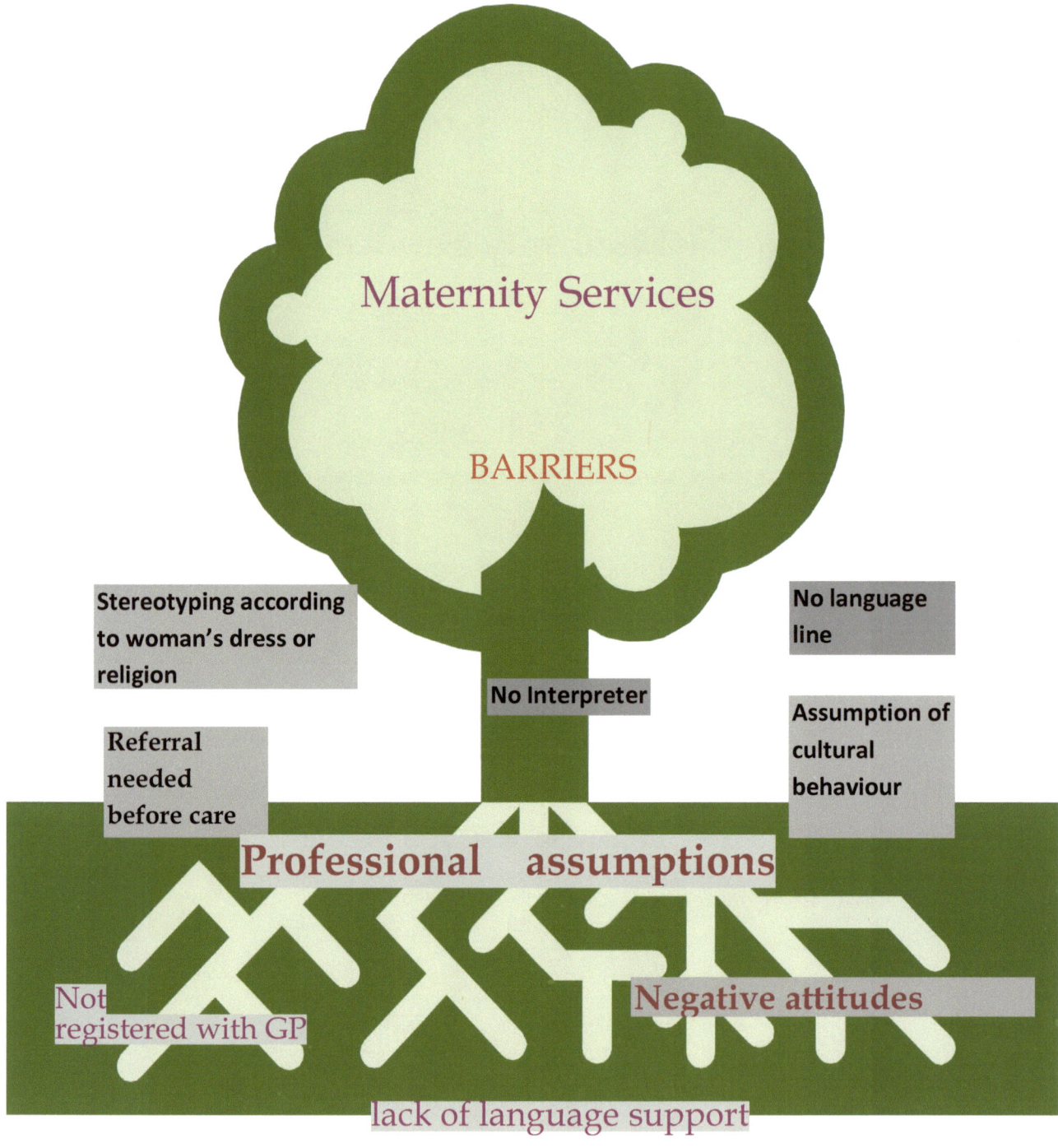

Adapted from MEDACT, Access to Maternity Services, Barriers created by health professionals and systems 2009

What steps can be taken to improve access?

Individual steps

Beware of language barriers, offer an interpreter at the first instance.

Never assume how a woman may behave if they are from a certain cultural background. Adopt the habit of asking pertinent questions about a woman's beliefs before planning care.

Be supportive and willing to discuss any cultural norms with the woman in a non-biased manner, for example the wearing of certain clothes, obeying rituals, need for chaperones, and discussion of sexual health with a male professional.

It would be useful to found out how pregnancy care is carried out in the woman's country of origin so that any misconceptions can be corrected.

Discuss with the woman how the healthcare system works in the UK, for example pattern of care, blood tests, seeing the GP etc.

Organisational steps

Adopting the use of culturally appropriate advice leaflets, maternity notes, for woman regarding pregnancy for example on diet, breastfeeding and postnatal care.

Cultural knowledge packs for health professionals available in ward areas as quick reference guides.

Adopting use of community centre to provide information on certain cultures as a regular occurrence. For example, training of new staff, devising of information packs for patients.

Use culture as the first point of assessment for the woman when devising care plans or patterns of care. This will allow consideration for acknowledging cultural norms or respecting any taboos.

How can cultural knowledge increase access to health services?

Helping African women to engage with healthcare services can be done by using culturally appropriate posters and literature to target particular groups. However, maintaining engagement with certain groups can be achieved by ensuring on contact that culturally sensitive care and advice is given. Creating an understanding with African women can be achieved by acknowledging cultural differences and at the same time facilitating woman's needs by removing barriers that may compromise their culture. The next sections will explore these cultural norms country by country and how they may create barriers to maternity care.

References

1. Hobbs, A. 2008 Africa, Sino publishing house, China.

2. Truter, L. 2007 African Traditional Healers, Cultural and religious beliefs intertwined in a holistic way, South African Pharmaceutical Journal, September, pp.56-60.

3. WHO 2001 Legal Status of Traditional medicine and Complementary/Alternative Medicine: A Worldwide review, Geneva, WHO.

4. Awoko Higginsbottom, G, M. 2000 Breastfeeding Experiences of Women of African Heritage in the United Kingdom, Journal of Transcultural Nursing, vol.11, no.1, pp.55-63.

5. Carolan, M. 2008 Antenatal care perceptions of pregnant African women attending maternity services in Melbourne, Australia, Midwifery, doi.10.1016, J.midwifery.2008.03.005.

6. CEMACH 2007 Saving Mother's Lives, Reviewing maternal death to make motherhood safer-2003-2005, CEMACH.

7. The Londoner 2005 Africans in London, April.

8. Office of National Statistics 2012 www.ons.gov.uk/dcp29904_291554.pdf

9. MEDACT, Breaking Down the Barriers, Module 3: Access to Maternity Services, www.medact.org accessed 3.6.2014.

Bibliography

Omonzejele, P. F. 2008 African Concepts of Health, Disease and Treatment:

An Ethical Inquiry, Explore, vol.4, no.2, pp.120-126.

Kubkeli P S. 2000 Traditional healing practices using medicinal herbs, The

Lancet, vol 354, pp.24.

Section two

WEST AFRICAN CULTURE

2.1 NIGERIAN CULTURE AND CHILDBIRTH

Nigeria is located in Africa its neighbouring countries are Benin to the east, Congo to the North and Cameroon to the west. The name of Nigeria is taken from the river Niger one of largest rivers in Nigeria. The population of Nigeria is approximately 173 million and is the second largest populated country in the world. There are over 200 ethnic groups in Nigeria, the largest of these being the Hausas in the north, the Yoruba's in the south and the Igbos (Ibos) in eastern Nigeria.

Language

Yoruba, Hausa and Ibo are the three main languages spoken in Nigeria. There are over 250 individual tribal languages. Hausa is the oldest known language in West Africa dating back to as early as the ninth century. English is spoken in educational institutes and used for business. Pidgin English, which is also spoken, is a mix of English and native languages.

Religions

Christianity, Islam and native tribal religions are practiced in Nigeria. Muslims mainly reside in the North of Nigeria. Native religion is the practice of worshipping deities, ancestors and tribal gods; this practice is spread throughout the country. Muslims and Christians may intertwine their beliefs with native beliefs. The most common Christian forms are Anglican, Methodists, Seventh - day Adventist and Jehovah's witnesses.

Society

Nigeria is a patriarchal and hierarchal society and men are considered to be the decision makers in all aspects of family life. It is not unusual to use the term 'Ma' to address a woman and alternatively 'Sir' to address a man. Elders are considered to be wise in all matters and are granted great respect. In social situations the most senior person has the responsibility of making decisions that are in the best interest of the family or social group. Extended families are still the norm and are the backbone of the social system; the family cares for all members. Although the extended family is becoming diminished in modern societies there are still strong links with family whether a person resides in Nigeria or the UK.

Communication

A person is usually greeted by using a handshake; however when greeting a woman allow her to extend her hand first. It is considered rude to rush a greeting, and time should be spent enquiring about a person's health before any general conversation. Nigerians do not usually practice a first name culture so one should ask for permission to use the first name. When addressing a person who is much older it is a sign of respect to bow the head or curtsey. Due to the various ethnic groups in Nigeria, communications styles may vary. Some individuals may use proverbs to enrich what they are saying. The Yoruba people often use humour to enhance their communication.

Nigerian's tend to speak more directly and loudly which someone from another culture may find unusual. A Nigerian person who feels passionately about a subject may become more emotional and use hand and facial expressions. Hand expressions may also be used if the individual feels distressed or disappointed.

Point to remember

It may be beneficial to be aware of these cultural norms in communication. This knowledge can assist in engaging with the woman.

Pregnancy

A woman's inclination to make decisions on health and reproductive issues may be influenced by the father, husband or son depending on the circumstances. Education also influences how much autonomy the woman has; other influences on her decisions are the woman's mother or her mother -in -law. The economic position of the woman may also affect her choices in childbearing. In Nigerian tradition it is forbidden to discuss and count the number of children, however economic problems, education and religious orientation mean that husbands and wives are more likely to discuss these issues. Childlessness is the most dreaded tragedy for a man or woman to experience in Nigeria's patriarchal society. The power of traditional values and the strong influence of family mean that cultural rituals are normally followed.

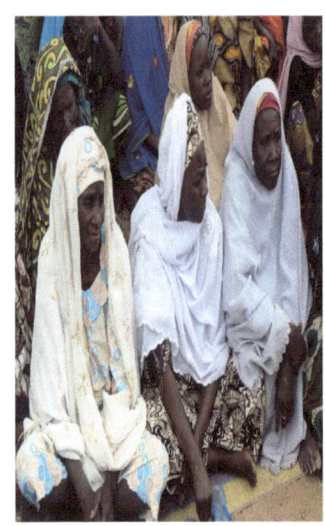

Point to remember

A woman may not attend for her booking appointment with her partner. This should not be seen as lack of partner support but as a cultural norm that men do not usually discuss women's reproductive issues.

Seeking treatment for health problems depends on cultural beliefs about the cause and cure of illnesses. Traditional medicine may still be used whether a woman resides in Nigeria or the UK.

There are various forms in which traditional medicine is administered, for example herbs may be boiled for bathing or drinking. A common Nigerian belief is the necessity to maintain a hot/ cold balance within the body. Blood is considered hot so a person who has experienced any blood loss is kept warm in order to restore the body's natural balance.

Antenatal

Pregnancy is normally confirmed either by cessation of menses or detection of fetal movements. This practice poses a problem as it may delay a woman from consulting her

GP. The pregnancy may not be considered to be 'settled' until well after 12 weeks in Nigerian culture. Pregnancy is seen as a normal bodily function needing treatment only when something goes wrong such as fever or oedema.

During pregnancy, to prevent harm, the woman may be encouraged not to go out alone at night. She is also encouraged not to fight or quarrel as this behaviour is thought to be harmful to the baby. A common Nigerian belief is that there is a presence of evil spirits and witches who can cause ill health or misfortune to individuals. Holy water is commonly used for protective and treatment purposes, for example prevention of miscarriage, indigestion, and prolonged labour and warding off any evil spirit. This holy water may be drank or rubbed all over the body. The woman's mother or mother- in - law normally counsels the woman on what procedure to follow. These procedures are also used to prevent harm to the baby. A woman's pregnancy is kept undisclosed and is only exposed to close family members to prevent the exposure to evil intentions. Walking and performing plenty of exercises are believed to prevent malpositions. Certain foods are taken or avoided during pregnancy and will be discussed in the next segment.

Cultural reasons why women may not seek health advice from professionals may be due to their lack of trust in healthcare services, unawareness of importance of antenatal care, financial difficulty or a fear that western medicine may harm their unborn child.

Point to remember

A woman may present late for pregnancy care for many reasons, however confirming the pregnancy and announcing it to the world is not done for fear of making an error or attracting evil spirits. She may not wish to make contact with healthcare services until she is sure that she is pregnant, which may be two to three missed menstrual cycles. This poses problems in achieving an antenatal booking at a recommended 8 to 10 weeks.

Diet

Nigerians combine traditional foods with western styles of food. Nigerian cuisine is based around staple foods eaten with stews or soups. Foods play an important role in all ceremonies such as marriages and naming ceremonies. Traditional Nigerian foods may be eaten by hand, however with western influences the use of knives and forks are common. It is considered unclean to use the left hand to eat.

Root staples are yam and cassava, and common meats are goat, beef and chicken. Fish (dried or fresh) and rice is very popular in Nigerian cuisine. Nigeria has plenty of tropical fruits including mangoes, bananas, pineapples, papayas and coconuts. Vegetables include okra (lady's fingers), spinach, melon seed and corn.

In Nigerian culture, biscuits cakes and sweets are not considered staple foodstuffs, but luxury items. However, western influences have increased the use of these types of foods. Bread is the only western food that is used as a food staple. Fruit is commonly used to break fasts in Muslim and Christian religions. The Nigerian diet is rich in meat and starchy foods, but only a small amount of green vegetables and dairy products consumed. Vegetables are normally overcooked reducing iron content.

A common traditional dish is vegetable soup and pounded yam/gari. The soup is made from various vegetables, assorted meats, okra, melon seeds, and oil. The pounded yam is boiled yam that has been mashed (pounded) and made into a dough. If pounded yam is not used then grounded cassava that has been dried (gari) is mixed with hot water and made into dough to eat with the soup. Jelloff rice is rice mixed with peppers, onions, tomatoes, oil and boiled to make a savoury dish, very similar to paella. Rice, fried plantain (dodo) and beans can be eaten with various soups or stews.

Food products that women use to help to maintain wellbeing

Egg and lots of vegetables are eaten during pregnancy, and women are advised not to drink iced water or alcohol, as this is not beneficial to the baby. To prevent nausea women chew native chalk, this is white in colour and can be found in the UK. Eating clay may also be used to help with pica. To relieve constipation women drink plenty of water, and vegetables. Fruit and vegetables are thought to cause Indigestion and prolonged labour and are eaten in small quantities.

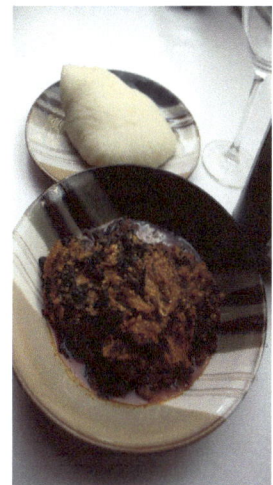

Point to remember

Having some knowledge of Nigerian traditional foods will assist the health professional to give appropriate dietary advice to the woman. It may also be helpful to be aware of any natural remedies, which women may use in pregnancy

The start of labour is normally kept a secret apart from informing immediate family members. Partners traditionally do not attend for labour and a trusted female friend or relative would normally escort the woman. With western influences this practice is changing.

Culturally food is not usually allowed in labour, even early labour as any consumption of food is believed to cause vomiting. To deal with contractions women are asked to mobilise and pain medication is avoided due to fear of harm to the baby. During the second stage of labour shouting is discouraged, as this period of labour is sacred in Western Nigeria. However, it is not unusual for the Nigerian woman to shout and click her fingers whilst in labour as a coping mechanism for dealing with pain.

Prolonged labour is viewed as a punishment for violating certain traditions or infidelity. A delay in labour may also be blamed on evil spirits bewitching the woman. There is a stigma attached to caesarean birth, as a woman may be seen in Nigerian culture as being incomplete for not giving birth vaginally.

Points to remember

Labour is considered a women's affair so do not be surprised if the woman's partner is not in attendance. In Nigeria a man would not normally be expected to be present at this time but a female companion. It is important not to pressurise partners to attend. A woman may ask her pastor or priest to attend to carry out certain prayers in order to prevent evil spirits causing a bad outcome of pregnancy.

Postnatal

The placenta traditionally in some tribes is buried in the garden or close to a fruit tree, which becomes the child tree. This may still be practiced in the UK. Some Nigerians believe that if the placenta is not disposed of correctly it may be eaten by an animal and cause a bad characteristic in the child. One belief is that if a rat eats the placenta the child will become a thief. A Nigerian mother may ask for their placenta so that they can dispose of it safely.

The baby

The new baby is welcomed with dancing and prayer immediately after delivery. Bathing the baby is done immediately; as it is believed that if not performed it may cause the baby to have body odour when older. It is important to remove any blood from the baby's head as this is seen as unclean.

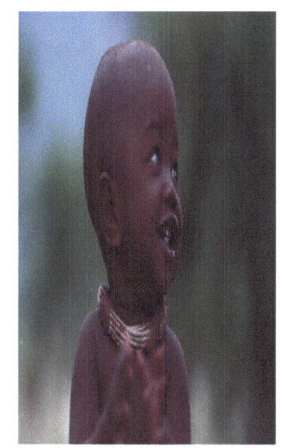

Zineflaz.blogspot.com

Some mothers may want to give water to the baby as a first feed, however, the baby is breast-fed as it is recognised that breast milk is beneficial to the baby. The baby not immediately be given a name, this occurs on the seventh or eight day.

Point to remember

It is important to explain the benefits of colostrum to the mother as she may wish to give a supplement to her baby at delivery.

The baby's cord is traditionally cared for by using herbs wrapped in a cloth, which is warmed and used to massage and press the cord; this is more commonly practiced in Western Nigeria. The midwife should be aware of the continuance of this practice and advise the mother of correct cord care. The first bath in some parts of Nigeria is performed using sand as a gentle abrasive then water and soap. In the Ibo culture the baby is massaged and thrown in the air to ensure limb straightness and to create fearlessness. The baby is not considered clean until all products of birth are removed including the vernix, which may take several days to disappear. The cord stump, which eventually drops of, is important, as this may be wanted by the mother for burial or praying before being discarded. Male circumcision is performed on the seventh day after birth in some tribes

Female genital cutting has now been more or less eradicated in Nigeria, but the health professionals should be aware that this may still be practised and inform the mother that it is an illegal practice. The baby may be carried on the mother's back secured by a broad cloth and fastened at the mother's breast.

Naming the baby is performed after the seventh day. There is usually a large ceremony/party with an abundance of food and drink. The aim of this ceremony is to present the baby to the world; this tradition is still practiced whether a woman resides in Nigeria or the UK. The names are normally sent from elders in Nigeria and can have various meanings normally acknowledging the circumstances around the birth. For example, if it has been a long awaited child the name could mean 'Thank you God' or 'At last you have come'.

The Mother

Immediately after birth the mother may not wish to hold her baby so the midwife should ask for her preferences. It is believed that the bodily fluids are unclean and a mother may want the baby to be dried first before having contact. Strict hand washing is adhered to in order to prevent infection or illness in the mother or baby. So you should allow her to wash her hands if she wishes to after delivery. The mother is encouraged to bathe as soon as possible after birth to remove the fluids of childbirth.

Older women of the Nigerian community normally perform daily ritualistic bathing and massaging of the mother's body with very hot water. This is to ensure well-being and reduce any aches and pains. The ritual of bathing is also a symbol of spiritual cleansing and may also be done by any female relatives or friends.

The lochia is seen as a necessary occurrence after birth, which is healthy and cleansing for the woman. Babies are nursed in heated rooms and kept very warm and the mother lies on a heated bed. This is within keeping with the hot/cold philosophy of traditional medicine health as the woman losing blood is considered to be losing heat.

The mother is asked to drink herbal remedies, which help to reduce after pains and lochia. She is encouraged to eat plenty of foods rich in calories, such as spicy soup and gruel enriched with salt and yam this is used to cleanse and involute the uterus. There is resting period traditionally observed where ample help is given to the new mother by her in- laws and family. The Nigerian belief is that these practices makes the woman stronger and enables her to regain her previous stamina.

Point to remember

In Nigerian culture the woman is normally looked after and supported by relatives and close family (mother and mother -in -law). This support system may not be available in the UK and may increase the risk of postnatal depression. It is important for health professionals to be aware of what support systems are available to women.

Bibliography

Culture of Nigeria, www.every culture.com/Ma-Ni/Nigeria.html. accessed 28.8.2014

Okafor, C. 2000 Folklore Linked to Pregnancy and Birth in Nigeria, Western Journal of Nursing Research, vol. 22, pp. 189.

Illiyasu, Z. Kabir, M. Galadanci H. S. Abubalar I. S. Salihu H. M Aliyu M.H .2006 Postpartum beliefs and practices in Danbare village, Northern Nigeria, Journal of Obstetrics and Gynaecology, vol. 26. no.3 pp. 211-215

Lawoyin, T. Olusheyi, O. C. Adewole D and L 2007 Men's Perception of Maternal Mortality in Nigeria , Journal of Public Health Policy, vol. 28, pp. 299-318.

2.2 GHANAIAN CULTURE AND CHILDBIRTH

Ghana is located in West Africa, with a population of approximately 20 million. Neighbouring countries are the Ivory Coast, Burkina Faso and Togo. Ghana was formally colonised by the British and was the first African country to gain independence from European rule.

Language

The national language in Ghana is English; there are over sixty indigenous languages. Akan (Twi) is the most widely spoken version and has acquired informal national status. Ga and Ewe are the next two major languages. Hausa may also be spoken as a trade language amongst people in the north of Ghana.

Religions

Christianity, Islam and traditional African religions have an equal amount of adherents. However, Christians and Muslims still follow some form of indigenous practice. Traditional beliefs vary between ethnic groups. In every tribal religion there is acknowledgement of spiritual beings, including ancestors and spirits. Ga people focus on the worshipping of priests of the ocean, inlets and lagoons.

Society

Most of Ghanaian ethnic groups are patrilineal apart from the Akan people who are mainly matrilineal. The majority of Ghanaians believe that marriage is a family matter, not just a contract between two individual persons. Marriage requires the approval of the family. Extended families are common however western influences and poor financial status have increased the number of nuclear families. Ghanaian's place great emphasis on politeness and formality. It is respectful to ask about a person's health and family on greeting. Visitors to a house are expected to greet each family member.

and great respect is attached to age and social status. A younger person should **always** show respect to an elder. The right hand is used to take objects or give objects from a person. English words such as silly, foolish or nonsense are highly offensive to some individuals.

Pregnancy

In Ghana cultural practices and beliefs are attached to childbirth, contraception and pregnancy. Some of these cultural practices are harmful such as dietary taboos. In Ghana a pregnancy may be considered viable at approximately 26 weeks. Until this time a woman may not announce the pregnancy to avoid harm or risk to her unborn child. Others become aware of a woman's condition as the pregnancy progresses and it becomes visible. Information and advice about pregnancy is normally obtained from elderly or experienced female family members.

Point to remember

A Ghanaian woman may have several reasons why she has not accessed maternity early on in pregnancy. It is important to discuss these issues with her in order to remove any misconceptions.

Diet

The Ghanaian diet consists of starchy staple eaten with soup or stew. The main carbohydrates are plantain, cassava, cocoyam (taro), corn (mainly Ga people), millet and rice. Fats in the Ghanaian diet are normally obtained from red palm or groundnut oil.

The main dairy product in the Ghanaian diet is milk. A popular traditional dish is called fufu, which is pounded plantain or tubers in combination with cassava, eaten with soup made with vegetables, meat or fish and hot peppers. Kenkey is another popular food staple in Ghana, it is made from fermented corn, which is rolled into dough balls and boiled in water. It is normally eaten with a spicy soup containing meat or stew.

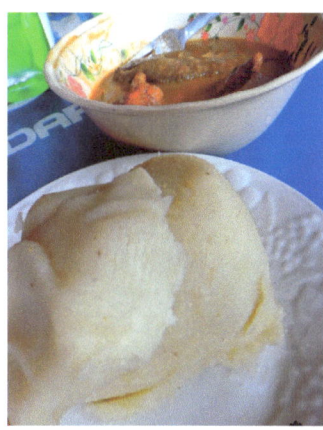

Common soups are made from palm nut or peanuts.

Foods that are rich in iron are plantains and spinach. Other vegetables eaten are tomatoes garden eggs and okra.
The main fruits are mangoes, papaya, oranges and pineapples.

Bread is a major European import and is eaten at breakfast.

Food products that women use to help to main wellbeing

To prevent nausea the woman may chew on a stick to alleviate symptoms. Eating red sand or white chalk is used to relieve pica. If the woman is constipated she is encouraged to drink plenty of water and eat oranges.

There is a belief that certain foods may cause oedema, proteinuria or premature labour. Preventing women from eating a well-balanced diet.

Point to remember

It is important to discuss common pregnancy ailments with the woman and discuss the causes of this. Misconceptions may prevent her from accessing medical care in a timely manner

Antenatal

There are certain taboos women adhere to, to prevent harm to the pregnancy. She may not go out late at night. The pregnancy is not discussed or mentioned to avoid unwanted attention. Fear of the unknown may prevent a pregnant woman from accessing hospital care, especially if she is used to having care from traditional sources. To ensure maternal well being she is encouraged not to eat late at night and to have plenty of rest. Massage is commonly used to prevent backache.

Labour

During labour sometimes the husband may be involved and be present at the delivery. However, it is more likely that a senior female family member will be present for support during this time. The woman is given warm water to drink to help with the pain of the contractions.

Postnatal

In Ghana the placenta is traditionally buried near the family home to prevent having a wayward child.

The baby

The baby after delivery is traditionally given water to assist with the passing of meconium. The woman's mother or a woman of the mother's choice will bathe baby and continue to bathe the baby each time until she can perform this chore by herself. Colostrum is considered unhealthy and expelled, however it is recognised that breastfeeding is beneficial and this is encouraged. Herbs may be applied to the umbilical cord to aid healing. Male circumcision is normally performed ideally on the seventh or eighth day.

The name of baby is normally given after approximately a week of age. It is thought that until this time the baby is a stranger from the ancestral world and may decide to return. The naming of a baby in Ghanaian culture is unique compared to anywhere else in the world. The baby is given two names one for the day of the week on which it was born. The other name is normally after an influential or good person, an ancestor or a name that has a religious meaning. Listed below are the names given to Ghanaians according to the day of the week on which they were born.

DAY OF THE WEEK	MALE	FEMALE
MONDAY	KOJO	ADJOA
TUESDAY	KWABENA	ABENA
WEDNESDAY	KWAKU	AKUA
THURSDAY	YAW	YAA
FRIDAY	KOFI	AFUA
SATURDAY	KWAME	AMA
SUNDAY	KWESI	AKOSUA

The mother

In Ghana forty days rest is considered important after delivery. The mother may go out before the seventh day but the baby is not taken out before this time unless it is necessary or in emergency situations. The mother is given herbs to eat mixed with meals, which is used to expel blood clots and improve lactation. Intercourse is

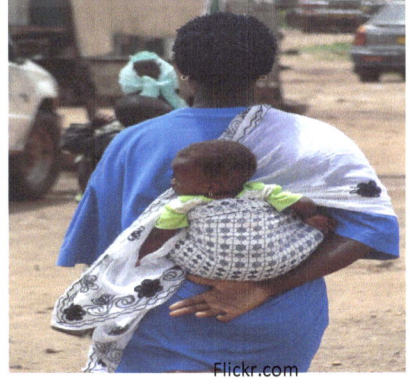
Flickr.com

traditionally forbidden in the postnatal period. To help expel the lochia and reduce bleeding, previously women were encouraged to use steam on the perineum. This practice is now phasing out with education.

Point to remember

Discuss with the woman any rituals that she finds important in the postnatal period. Give reason for avoiding harmful rituals to the woman.

Bibliography

Bansah, M. O'Brien, B. Oware-Gyekye, M.N. 2007 Perceived prenatal learning needs of multigravid Ghanaian women, Midwifery, doi:10.1016/J.midw.2007.07.06.

Nyinah, S. 1997 World Health, vol. 50, no.2, pp22-3.

Culture of Ghana, www.every culture.com/Ge-it/Ghana.html, accessed 28.8.2014

Section three

EAST AFRICAN CULTURE

3.1 SOMALIAN CULTURE AND CHILDBIRTH

Somalia is located in East Africa, which is commonly known as the horn of Africa. Neighbouring countries are Ethiopia, Djibouti and Kenya. Somalia means milk, a name chosen by the people to represent their nomadic farming tradition. Somalis are the only people of Arab African ethnicity and they are a clan-based nation. The British mainly colonised the north of Somalia, whilst the French and Italians colonised the South. There are many Kenyans who claim to be ethnic Somalians as they migrated from Somalia in colonial times and were trapped behind closed borders after decolonisation. Many Somali's are nomadic or have come from a nomadic culture. In 1991 a civil war erupted in Somalia causing mass migration to neighbouring countries, the United States and Europe.

The four main ethnic groups in Somalia are the Hawiye, Darod and Rahanwayn in the south and the Isaq in the north. The Hawiye and the Darod are the two largest ethnic groups. The Bantu is a term used in Somalia to describe people in Somalia of Kenyan origin and they make up less than 15% of the population. Somali's also live in Kenya, Ethiopia and Djibouti.

Languages

Somali is the common language taught spoken by all Somalians, Arabic is also spoken due the Koran being written in this language. A Somali may often understand Arabic even if they do not speak the language. In schools Somali and Arabic are the two compulsory languages, and English, French or Italian may also be taught. Not all girls go to school past primary age, but Arabic is taught at this stage. Somali did not become a written language until 1973. Literacy in Somalia has dropped from 80% to 30% due to poor educational services.

Religions

The main religion in Somalia is Islam; approximately 90% are Sunni Muslims of the Shafi'ite rite, with interest in Sufi spiritualism. This is characterised by chanting, whirling and chewing quat (a narcotic lead). There is a very small percentage of Christianity practiced by workers or families who in the past had lived in Europe or other African countries. Muslims must pray five prescribed times a day for an average of five to ten minutes. These times are fixed at noon, mid afternoon, sunset, early evening and 6am. Ablution is made before prayer. This involves washing the face arms and legs and the private parts. Muslims also prefer to wash with water after a bowel movement and the left hand is always used for washing.

The two main Somalian holidays are Eid-al fitr end of Ramadan and occurs in the ninth month of the Islamic calendar. Fasting is performed from dawn to sunset. Pregnant women, nursing mothers, the ill and children are exempt from fasting. However, some women may not adhere to this and continue to fast although they are pregnant or nursing. The second Muslim holiday is the 10th day of the last month of the Islamic calendar. These dates can vary from year to year.

Point to remember

Ramadan is a very important Muslim festival. Pregnant women may continue to fast even though it is not required in the Koran in pregnancy. Sensitivity is needed when discussing the importance of not fasting in pregnancy.

Society

The Islamic belief affects all aspects of Somali culture. The family does not just consist of blood relatives but anyone who lives together. Children are given a revered position as they are important for the future and welfare of the extended family. Elders are respected even if they are strangers to the family. A Somali woman often lives with her husband's family; she will however keep her family name. Hence, a woman may have a different surname to her husband. Somali culture is male centered in public places although at home this may not be the case. After puberty boys and girls are forbidden to have any physical contract and handshakes are permitted only between people of the same sex. The right hand is considered clean and is used for handshaking and eating. Clans are mainly patrilineal but families can be egalitarian in their nature. The culture affects every aspect of Somali life, how to eat, how to greet, how to respect others and how to respond in any given situation. There is no word for please in the Somali language, hence people in the UK may find the lack of use of this word discourteous.

Birthdays are not particularly celebrated in Somalia and individuals may not know their exact date of birth. Normally birth dates are rounded off to the nearest year. On the other hand, anniversaries of a person's death are noted and celebrated.

Dress

Islamic tradition influences the type of dress women wear. Women must wear the Hijab, which is a form of dress that covers the whole body except the face. She starts dressing this way from the age of seven

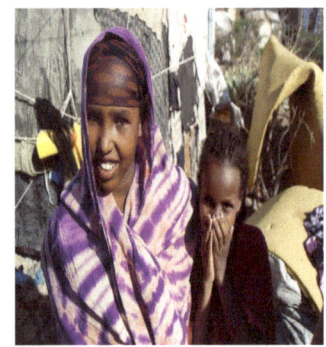

Flickr.com

Pregnancy

Somalian families are usually large in number ranging from six to eight children. This is considered an ideal family size. Contraception and abortion are taboo matters to most Somalis, due to their strong Muslim belief that every pregnancy is a blessing from Allah and should not be interfered with. Childbearing is approached in a fatalistic and pragmatic way and every eventuality is considered Allah's will. Somali women find it difficult to talk about sexuality and may find the openness around sexuality in the UK strange. In Somalia women go to a hospital to see a specialist so may not be used to the idea of a GP. A Somali woman will expect to be asked for the whole of her medical history so that a correct diagnosis may be made. If this is not done then she may doubt the doctor's ability to treat their problem and may refrain from re attending or seek advice from elsewhere. Somalian's are verbal people and prefer to have treatments or medications explained to them verbally rather than being given a leaflet to read. Other factors that Somali's find important are open-mindedness, patience and non-judgmental inquisitiveness about Somalian culture.

In Somalia, herbal medicines are used for varying disorders such as colds, haemmorhoids, diabetes and high blood pressure. These are normally fresh herbs which women may be able to access in the UK. Koranic cures are also used, whereby family members read verses from the Koran to the ill person. Somali's believe that an admirer or jealous person may use the evil eye to cause ill health in the recipient. An example of this is a health professional telling a woman that her baby is big and healthy. The mother fears this praise as it may result in harm to the baby.

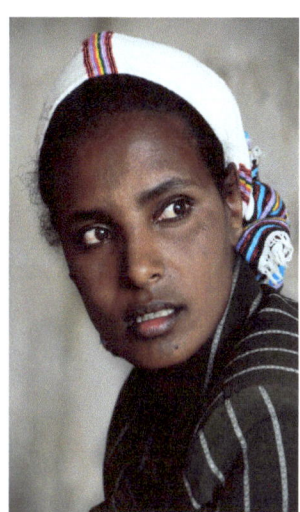

Antenatal

Pregnancy is normally recognised when the woman is in her 12th week and this is when she will seek medical advice. It is not usually done earlier for fear of a false pregnancy; however, the woman may tell her husband. This is significant, as women will tend to present late to their GP for pregnancy care. Once pregnancy is confirmed a woman may approach a Muslim sheik to write some verses from the Koran on a piece of paper that she folds and wear about her body. This is to prevent harm to the pregnancy, although it is not written in the Koran that this is necessary or approved of by the faith, traditionally this practice may still persist.

Advice about the pregnancy is normally obtained from elder women in the family, however due to living in the UK this is practice is not always possible. Somali women will seek advice from her GP but if this is a man and there are language barriers she may not feel comfortable talking about intimate problems. Due to the language barrier she would usually attend appointments with her husband. If there is no one who can interpret for her then this will delay her going to the GP.

A health professional should not assume that the Somali woman has knowledge of reproductive health and anatomy. In Somalia there is a culture of strict sexual modesty and taboo in discussing sexual topics.

Point to remember

A Somali woman will normally attend appointments with her husband or a person who can speak English. A language barrier may be the main reason why she may not be able to attend appointments so the health professional should be aware of this and offer an interpreter.

Diet

The Somali diet is governed by the Muslim practice that all foods consumed must be Halal. This is any food of plant origin or animal origin that conforms to the religious method of slaughtering. Forbidden foods (haram) are foods not slaughtered in the correct way, including pork , alcohol, blood and foods containing any ingredients from haram foods. The main staple in the Somali diet is semolina, which is made into a

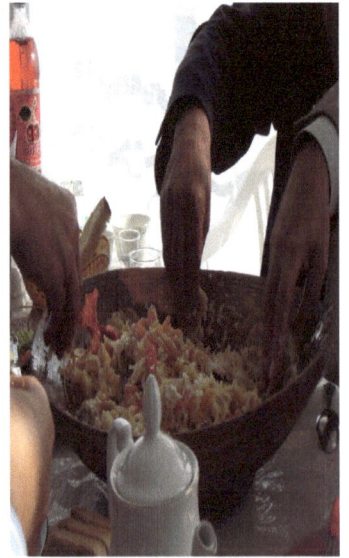

paste and eaten with a spicy meat and vegetable dish.

Anjero is a maize based pancake, eaten at breakfast, which is also used to eat meat or vegetable stew. Another common dish is Iskudhexkaris a meal cooked in the pot, a mixture of rice vegetables and meats, a popular Somalian dish. Lamb or goat's meat is popular in Somalian cuisine but fish is not generally liked. Tea is a popular drink, drunk 4-6 times a day with plenty of sugar.

Some Somalis are fond of spaghetti or macaroni due to the previous Italian influences during colonisation. Somalis eat many vegetables such as broccoli, peas, potatoes, and green leafy vegetables such as spinach. However, the normal Somali culture is to overcook these vegetables, which destroys all the nutrients. Frying of food is the most common cooking method in Somalia.

There are no particular foods that Somali women are asked to avoid in pregnancy which mean midwives have to be specific in ensuring that women understand the importance of avoiding foods that are contraindicated in pregnancy.

During Ramadan, some women may continue to fast despite being pregnant, it is important to explain the possible detrimental effects fasting can have on the mother and unborn fetus. Ultimately, it is the mother's decision if she continues to fast and her decision has to be respected. Some Somali women may also limit their food intake to control the size of their baby; this practice is common amongst women who have undergone female genital cutting (FGC).

Food products that women may use to help maintain well-being

Liver, which is contraindicated in pregnancy due to high levels of vitamin A is eaten in Somalia to prevent anaemia. Sour oranges or mud from the ground is used to help with pica. Boiled water from millet husk is added to milk and yoghurt to relieve constipation.

Point to remember

Discuss with the woman the best diet to meet her nutritional and cultural needs, and be aware of any foods that are culturally eaten that are contraindicated in pregnancy.

Labour

In Somalia, it is forbidden for men to be present during labour, however in the UK this practice may not be adopted. Men prefer for a female relative to be present, so a husband may escort his wife to the hospital and only stay if there is no available female who can attend. Nearly all mothers will have been infibulated, a form of female genital cutting (FGC), which involves the cutting of the vaginal labia and clitoris and closing these so that only a small opening is left for the purpose of menses and urination (Gudnin ka nagaha). This may pose a problem particularly if there is keloid formation or the vulval tissue is rigid. At delivery there is increased risk of perineal lacerations and the need for an episiotomy.

Point to remember

It is vital to inform women that in the UK it is illegal to reinfibulate after delivery. Somalia women may be too shy to talk about FGC, as it is acknowledged in the western world that it is a barbaric practice.

It is essential to treat women with understanding and to use a non-judgmental attitude in order to engage with them during pregnancy and labour.

Food is not normally given to a Somali woman in labour so as not to cause nausea. To keep her energy levels elevated she may be given water with sugar added, or glucose. Women prefer to stand, lie or squat for first and second stage of labour. Massage using olive or almond oil may also be performed by female attendants. Somali women prefer not to take any pain relief for fear that it may harm the baby. Epidurals are particularly feared due to a believed risk of paralysis.

A Somali woman may refuse induction of labour for fear of damage to the baby, it is important for the midwife to counsel the women on the importance of induction of labour and the need for the women to still attend for an antenatal check even if she is declining induction. It is believed in the Somali culture that the baby should initiate labour and it will come when it is ready. Somali women also fear caesarean section as it is felt that the operation may prevent future pregnancies or cause infirmity.

Points to remember

It is important when offering the Somali women pain relief to emphasize the safety of any medications. The midwife should be aware that a woman might refuse such medication if her husband is not present, as she may need to seek his approval. FGC is a sensitive issue for Somali women and health professionals should be aware of this particularly if the woman is in labour. It is essential to discuss with the woman at booking the type of female genital cutting she has, in order to arrange appropriate care in the antenatal and labour periods.

Postnatal

The baby is welcomed into the world by ritual prayer spoken by the father who faces towards Mecca. The baby should be cleaned of any blood immediately after delivery.

The baby

The Muslim call to prayer or adhaan ("God is great, there is no God but Allah. Muhammad is the messenger of Allah. Come to prayer.") are the first words a newborn Muslim baby should hear. His or her father whispers them into the right ear of the child. The baby's first taste should be something sweet, so parents may use honey or chew a piece of date and rub the juice along the baby's gums. It was a practice carried out by the Prophet Mohammed (pbuh) and is believed to help small digestive systems to kick in.

Breastfeeding is the normal practice for Somali women, and is performed for a period of two years or longer. It is believed that colostrum is harmful to the baby and it is preferred that baby's receive a supplement for the first 24-48 hours. Somali women believe that breast milk is insufficient in this period and will prevent a normal and healthy baby.

The baby in some ethnic Somali groups wears a bracelet made of an herb called malmal, to ward of the evil eye. This herb is not usually found in the UK but may be sent from Somalia. This same herb is traditionally attached to the umbilical cord for up to one week after birth. It is also common due to western influences to use antiseptics on the cord hence, it is important to educate the mother on the benefits of not using these. Other infant care practices are numerous warm baths and massages. Male circumcision is compulsory in Somali culture.

The baby is normally named on the 7th day with a name given by the Muslim sheikh, however in modern times this may not be practiced and the mother may name the child herself. The name is in general an Islamic name. The newborn baby is not generally taken out before seven days, as it is felt that before this time exposure to the outside environment is harmful to the baby.

Point to remember

Health professionals should be sensitive and ensure that the woman and her family are given time to perform the religious rituals after the birth of the baby.

The mother

Somali women are also expected to stay in the home for seven days and abstain from sexual intercourse for 40 days according to the Koran. This is known as afatanbah. Traditionally she is not expected to prepare food if she is still bleeding and may employ assistance from female relatives for this purpose. The mother is given meals of broth, which is made with meat and vegetables; this is used to aid lactation. In the following days tea with plenty of milk is taken to increase milk supply.

A barrier method is the common form of contraception used (condoms) and the practice of breastfeeding is believed to prevent another pregnancy. A cloth may be used to tie around the woman's abdomen in the postnatal period to aid evolution of the uterus. Some Somali women may still practice a tradition of using herbs and an incense called 'dush' to tighten the vaginal orifice and to create a pleasant smell.

Point to remember

Breastfeeding is the main form of contraception used in Somali women and it is important to inform the woman that this method is not 100% effective.

Bibliography

Berggren, V. Bergstrom, S. Edberg, A. 2006 Being Different and Vulnerable: Experiences of Immigrant African Women Who Have Been Circumcised and Sought Maternity Care in Sweden, Journal of Transcultural Nursing, vol.17 pp. 50- 57.

Carroll, J. Epstein, R. Fiscella, K. Gipson, T. Volpe, E. Pascal, J. 2007 Caring for Somali women: Implications for clinician-patient communication, Patient Education and Counselling, vol. 66, pp.337-345.

Small, R. Gagnon, A. Gissler, M. Zeitlin, J. Glazier, RH. Haelterman, E. Martens, G. McDermot S. Urquia, M. Vangen S. 2008 Somali women and their pregnancy outcomes postmigration: data from six receiving countries, British Journal of Obstetricians and Gynaecologists, vol. 115, pp. 1630-1640.

Straus, L. McEwen, A. Mohamed Hussein, F. 2009 Somali women's experience of childbirth in the UK: Perspectives from Somali health workers, Midwifery, vol. 25, pp. 181-186.

3.2 KENYAN CULTURE AND CHILDBIRTH

Kenya is located in East Africa and borders Somalia to the northeast, Ethiopia to the north, Sudan to the northwest, Uganda to the west, Tanzania to the south, and the Indian Ocean to the east. Kenya's population is approximately over thirty million. The main and most westernised tribe is the Bantu speaking Kikiyu (21%) of central Kenya who migrated from western Africa. The Nilotic people are the next largest tribe originating from Sudan. The Hamitic groups are mainly pastoral tribes from Ethiopia and Somalia. The other tribes are the Meru (5%), Kalenjin, Luyha, Luo (14%), Kisii, Kamba, Swahili, Masai and the Turkana.

Language

The official languages in Kenya are English and Kiswahili (or Swahili), which comes from the Arabic word meaning "coast," and is a mix of Arabic and Bantu, an African language. There are over forty native languages; English and Swahili are spoken in schools.

Religion

Christianity is the main religion and is practiced by approximately 70% of the population. Traditional religions are also practiced in Kenya. There is a small population of Kenyans living by the coast side who practice Islam. Many Kenyans believe in a supreme being and other spirits that are a part of every day life. For example, the Kikiyu believe that there is a spirit that controls crops and trees.

Society

The most significant events in Kenyan society are death and childbirth. Family loyalty and traditional beliefs hold strong in many communities. Rites of passage, especially initiation and marriage, remain very important and widely celebrated events. Families may consist of nuclear families that live close to each other. Cousins may call each other brother or sister and aunts and uncles may be called mother and father. Kenya is a patrilineal society and any children born during marriage belong to the father's family.

The birth of the first child proves a mother's womanhood. Kenyans believe in the after life and give great reverence to deceased ancestors, and individuals are only really considered dead if people fail to remember them. Marriage is an important event in Kenya because an individual can begin to establish his or her own kinship network.

Diet

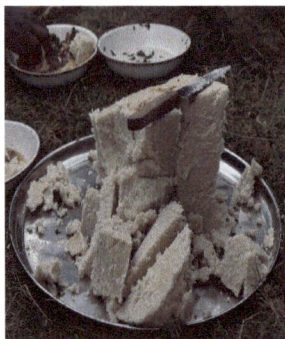

Corn (or maize) is the staple food of Kenyans. It is ground into flour and prepared as a porridge called posho or ugali which is sometimes mixed with mashed beans, potatoes, and vegetables, to make a dish called irio. This dish is rich in carbohydrates.. Common side dishes rich in iron are mboga, which is boiled greens and a banana porridge, called matoke.

Soup, mainly broth is eaten as well as curried stew called Githeri. A common drink called Chai is tea, mixed with milk ginger and sugar. Fruits popular in Kenya are mangoes, papaya, passion fruit, bananas and custard apples.

Foods mothers may avoid to maintain maternal well-being

During the last stages of pregnancy a woman may be forbidden to eat fatty foods and beans. A particular type of soil may be consumed which is believed to strengthen the body of the unborn child.

Antenatal

There are various traditions followed by Kenyan women whilst they are pregnant. Some mothers may not view a dead body, as it is feared that spirits will interfere with the pregnancy. Sexual activities are avoided during pregnancy to prevent the child being born with a disability. The husband is advised to even sleep in a different room from his wife during the latter stages of pregnancy. In some tribes the man is not allowed to have contact with his expectant wife if he is coming from outside into the house, until he has showered to prevent miscarriage. A Kenyan woman may belief that modern medicine is only necessary when things are going wrong.

> ## Point to remember
>
> It is important to discuss with the mother common beliefs that may prevent her from adhering to advice in pregnancy.

Labour

Traditionally Kenyan men are not involved in the birth process. In western society men are more inclined to attend with their wives in labour so this cultural norm is changing.

Postnatal

The baby

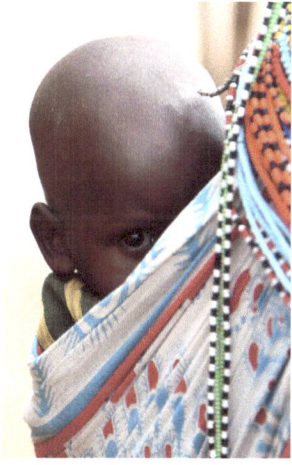

The name of the child is given depending on the season in which it is born, time of birth or whether it resembles or has the mark of a departed person. In one tribe whilst a child is crying, several names are called out and the child is named if it stops crying at a particular name. In the Meru tribe the child is named after the first animal its parents see. The Kenyan child is shielded from the evil eye, in the Kisii tribe this is done by using a red cloth. All male children are circumcised and in some tribes the parents may not have sexual intercourse until the circumcision is healed.

The mother

The cultural practice is to protect the mother and baby from any harm for up one month by ensuring she stays in the house. The mother is advised to keep breastfeeding as a method of contraception.

Bibliography

Bogaert, K. Ogunbanjo, G. A. 2008 Post-birth Rituals: Ethics and the Law, South African Family Practice, vol.50, no.2, pp.45-46.

Kamba Society, www.bluegecko.org/kenya/tribes/kamba/society.htm accessed 22.9.2014

Kenya: language, Culture, Customs and Etiquette, http:/www.kwintessential.co.uk/resources/global-etiquette/Kenya.html accessed 28.9.2014

Kikuyu-Introduction,www.bluegecko.org/kenya/tribes/kikuyu/index.htm accessed 22.9.2014

Magadi, M. A. Madise, N. J. Rodrigues R N. 2000 Frequency and timing of antenatal care in Kenya: explaining the variations between women of different communities, Social Science and Medicine, vol.51, pp.551-561.

Mosula, M. Asego, N. 2007 Kenyan Childbirth-The Many Myths and Taboos, The Standard, 1st October.

3.3 UGANDAN CULTURE AND CHILDBIRTH

Uganda is situated in east Africa situated between Kenya and The republic of Congo in East Africa. There are 17 tribes belonging to the Bantu and Nilotic tribes. The Baganda is the largest ethnic group and accounts for 17 % of the population. The second largest ethnic group is the Basoga which account for about 8 % of the population, the Bagisu constitutes roughly 5 % of the population. Up until the late 1960's there were over 70,000 people of Asian origin living in Uganda who were forced to leave the country by the then leader Idi Amin.

Language

Luganda is the native tongue spoken in Uganda and is the main national language. Languages that are spoken in educational institutes are English, Swahili and Luganda. Swahili has been approved as the country's second official language.

Religion

85% of the population is Christian whilst the remainder practice Islam and indigenous religions. The people of Uganda have adopted the shared practice of these religions . There is still a practice of western beliefs, traditional beliefs and belief in witchcraft and spirits.

Society

Family decision making is a male prerogative. Mother's in law particularly play an important role regarding making health decisions. Issues around childcare and food are women's concerns. However, the male person whether he is the father, son or brother of the woman has control over family issues and are the main decision makers.

Pregnancy

Having children in Ugandan culture is of the utmost importance whether the woman is married or unmarried, religious or not. Pregnancy is supposed to prepare the woman for the battle of labour and it is expected to be hard. Surviving pregnancy genders great respect as the woman has come through a hard battle. Dying in childbirth is considered a weakness; hence women who have survived childbirth are highly respected.

Sickness or death of an expecting mother is considered a normal and natural phenomenon.

Diet

The main food staple in Uganda is a starch maize meal called Ugali. This is normally eaten with a stew made with fish, chicken or meat. The stew may also be made with groundnut or beans. The common greens consist of amaranth (dodo), spinach and cabbage. Other vegetables eaten are yams, cassava and sweet potatoes. Fruits commonly eaten are bananas, mangoes, pawpaw, oranges and pineapples. Dairy dietary products consist of milk and gee.

Foods products that women may use to help to maintain wellbeing

For nausea and pica women may take herbs mixed with clay. An herbal concoction called emumbwa may be taken orally throughout pregnancy for fetal well being. Herbs are also used to make pelvic bones flexible thus preventing the need for caesarean section. Other herbs may be used to aid indigestion.

Antenatal

Once pregnant, the woman is not supposed to tell anyone except the father. This is apparently to lessen the chance of someone "bewitching" the woman and hurting the unborn child. A woman may fear to seek help from health professionals for fear of influence from witch doctors. Therefore, Ugandans find it somewhat rude if someone comment on someone else's pregnancy, or ask questions about it (Do you know the gender? When is the baby due?) questions. There is also a fear of preparing for the newborn whose viability is uncertain.

Only severe complications may be thought necessary for medical attention. Mild manifestations of fever, vomiting and oedema may be tolerated. Hence, women are not expected to report these ailments.

Point to remember

If the cultural norm is to expect pregnancy to be hard and difficult, please remind the woman that even minor ailments in pregnancy need to be taken heed off. If she is unsure she should always seek medical advice.

Labour

Traditionally kneeling down is the position used in labour. Expression of pain is a normal occurrence in labour. This expression is traditionally a part of a woman's upbringing to express pain as part and parcel of childbirth. It is also used to help to disconnect women from the pain of childbirth. Massage is used to help to alleviate pain and hasten the birth process. Men are not expected to be present in the labour room. Eating and drinking is encouraged.

Postnatal
The baby

Babies are believed to be born dirty with a bad smell, so the baby is required to be bathed after delivery. A bath is also believed to make the baby feel more comfortable and prevent any infection. Soapy or salty water is used for bathing. The cord is cared for using powder, spirit or herbs. Fast healing of the cord is believed to stop the after pains in the mother. If the cord has not fallen off then the baby is kept indoors. Breastfeeding is encouraged, although colostrum is considered to be bad for the baby.

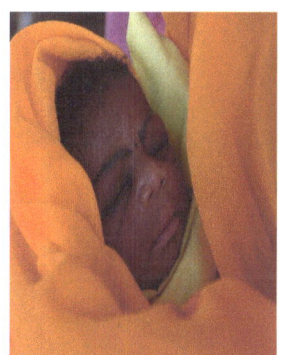

Flickr.com

Point to remember

Bathing the baby is a cultural norm which is harmless to the baby. Ensuring that the baby is kept warm during the bath is more important than trying to prevent the mother following this cultural norm.

The mother

In some parts of Uganda husbands observe a period of sexual abstinence, as the semen is believed to contaminate the mother's breast milk which may in turn affect the baby's health. However, in other parts of Uganda early sexual intercourse is encouraged in the belief that the semen will aid healing of any lacerations or perineal tears.

So, it can be seen that practices do vary according to tribal group. It is important to be aware of these taboos as this may prevent the mother from breastfeeding, resulting in her offering the baby alternative milk.

Bibliography

Bantebya Kyomuhendo, G. 2003 Low use of Rural Maternity Services in Uganda: Impact of Women's status, Traditional beliefs and Limited Resources, Reproductive Health Issues, vo.11, no.21, pp.16-26.

Odar, E. Wandabwa, J. Kiondo, P 2003 'Sexual practices of women within six months of childbirth in Mulago hospital, Uganda', African health Sciences, vol.3, no.3, pp. 117-123.

Waiswa, P. Kemigisa, M. Kiguli, J. Naikoba, S. Pariyo, G.W, Peterson, S. 2008 'Acceptability of evidenced-based neonatal care practices in rural Uganda-implications for programming' BMC Pregnancy and Childbirth vol.8, no.21, doi:10.1186/1471-2393.

Section four

SOUTHERN AFRICAN CULTURE

4.1 MALAWI

Malawi is a small country in the centre of southern Africa known as the warm heart of Africa. Its neighbouring countries are Tanzania, Zambia and Mozambique. The name Malawi comes from the Maravi, Bantu people who migrated from southern Congo. Malawi is one of the world's poorest countries and has few natural resources. It has a population of about 14.3 million with 90% of the population living in the rural areas, and a population growth rate of 1.57% (1999 est.). Malawi is divided into 28 districts, which have different cultural beliefs. Ethnic groups in Malawi are the Chewa, Nyanja, Yao, Tumbuka, Lomwe, Sena, Tonga, Ngoni, Ngonde, Asian and Europeans.

Languages

English is the official language in Malawi and is very widely spoken, particularly in main towns, but sometimes also in remote rural areas. Chichewa, is the common national tongue widely used throughout the country from 1968 until recently, it has served as the national language.

Religion

The Chewa people, who form the largest part of the population, are predominantly Christian/Protestant and the Yao people are mainly Muslims.

Society

Malawians are warm and friendly people who treat guests in revered manner. Showing hospitality to guests is a maintained Malawian culture.

Diet

The staple diet is Nshima, which is white maize; it can be eaten with Ndiwo a dish that contains onions, tomatoes, green vegetable and cassava or on occasion fish or meat.

Other Malawian staples are rice or potatoes. Starch is used as a relish and to give flavour to food. Common vegetables are cassava leaves, sweet potato leaves, bean leaves, pumpkin leaves, cabbage leaves and kale leaves. Popular fruits are guava, oranges, mangoes and bananas. Malawian's generally eat a diet rich in carbohydrates with small amounts of vegetables and fruits.

Foods that women may avoid to maintain well-being

It is believed that whilst pregnant a mother should not eat food that is cooked or prepared for example at a party or at a fast food restaurant. This is to prevent the possible consumption of foods prepared by a menstruating woman or by someone who has experienced a recent loss. It is believed that this contact will cause miscarriage or pregnancy loss.

Pregnancy

Childbearing women are seen as unique beings with physical, psychological, social and spiritual needs. Traditionally the woman's mother makes decisions about pregnancy care, in recent times these decisions are made by the father of the baby. However, once the woman becomes pregnant this is a woman's affair. Pregnant

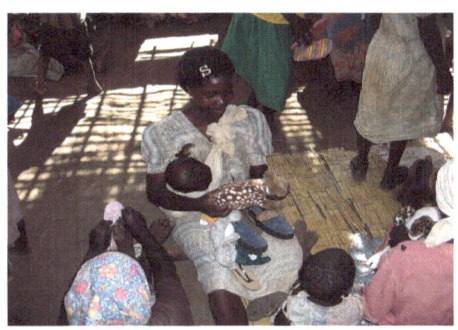

Malawian women rarely make these decisions by themselves as this raises the suspicion that the child does not belong to the husband/partner. The father decides family size and a large family is favoured with about six to eight children.

Antenatal

Pregnant woman in the Malawian culture should refrain from taking bitter medicine (modern or traditional) to avoid stillbirth or miscarriage. A pregnant woman should not have any contact with a dead person or attend a funeral for fear of miscarriage, preterm birth or death. Pregnant women should avoid quarrelling with people, which may give witches the opportunity to cause harm. To prevent miscarriage a woman may wear a string made from medicinal plants around the waist, which is only removed at the start of labour.

> ## Point to remember
>
> A Malawian may particularly refrain from taking medicines that are bitter, an explanation is needed of the importance of treatment.

Cessation of sexual activity is advised from the seventh month to prevent excess vernix in the baby. The buying and preparation of baby's clothes before the birth is not recommended as this may consequently lead to stillbirth. To prevent prolonged labour the Malawian women avoids standing in open doorways or peeping through windows as this is thought to cause the baby to become stuck in the birth canal. Towards the end of pregnancy the woman's mother or mother- in -law may stay with her to help with household chores.

Labour

Husband's attendance in labour rarely occurs in Malawi, mothers, aunts and mother- in-laws usually attend. Women are advised not to cry out in labour as this is considered disgraceful to her family and cultural group. Porridge mixed with Chibwaka (sweet potato) or raw eggs is given to the woman to eat as it is thought to have oxytocic properties.

Postnatal

The placenta after delivery may be asked for so that it can be disposed of correctly. It is normally buried with the maternal side up to prevent secondary infertility.

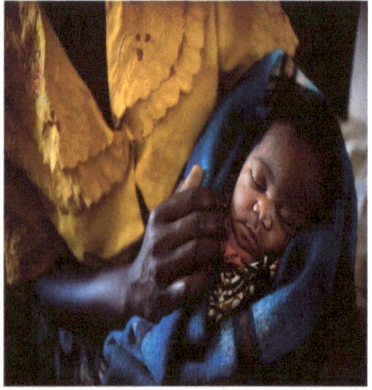

briantropiano.wordpress.com

The baby

The baby is kept indoors until the cord drops off and is not named until this time. After this time the baby is bathed in cold water with medicinal herbs. The cord may be treated with ashes. This is practice is a potential source of infection for the baby and may still be conducted in the UK. Breastfeeding is encouraged but again mixed feeding may occur. In addition, other foods may be given, as well as herbal infusion to prevent illness. The mother should be made aware of the dangers of this practice.

The mother

The woman is considered dirty if she is still losing lochia and up to one to two months after delivery. During this time she is not allowed to cook or have sexual intercourse. Once lochia has ceased she donates the clothes she has worn during this period. The principle of remaining in doors and keeping room may be followed similar to other African cultures.

Bibliography

Tolhurst, R. Theobald, S. Kayira, E. Ntonya, C. Kafulafula, G. Nielson, J. Broek, N. 2008 'I don't want all my babies to go to the grave":perceptions of preterm birth in Southern Malawi, Midwifery, vol.24, pp.83-98.

Gennaro, S. Kamwendo, L.A. Mbweza, E. Kersh Baumer R. 1997 Childbearing in Malawi. Africa, Journal of Obstetric, Gynaecologic and Neonatal Nursing, vol.27, no.22, pp.191-196.

4.2 ZIMBABWEAN CULTURE AND CHILDBIRTH

Zimbabwe is located in Southern Africa; surrounding countries are Botswana to the southwest, Mozambique to the east, Zambia to the northwest and South Africa to the south. The people of Zimbabwe are made up of several tribes which were derived from the Bantu people who migrated from the north of Africa to the south.

Language

English is the main language spoken in Zimbabwe and is taught in all schools.

The Mashona tribe is the largest tribe in Zimbabwe constituting 75% of the population. The language spoken by the Mashona tribe is Shona. The Matabele tribe constitutes 20% of the population and their dialect is Ndebele.

Religion

A majority of Zimbabweans are Christians although they continue to practice indigenous religions which involve communicating with spirits of the dead. In periods of ill health even devout Christians may abandon their religious beliefs to seek indigenous methods.

Society

Traditionally, the Zimbabwean family structure was extended; however' due to the change in the economic infrastructure this has begun to change. Women are beginning to become the leaders of family groups, although patriarchy is still very dominant in many family groups. These changes are mainly due to the increased educational status of women and western influences. A woman's social recognition can be affected by the fact that she is not married or childless. This may affect even friendships between women. Being loyal to ones husband, family or kinship is paramount in Zimbabwean culture. The Shona culture have many taboos which are used to control the activities of it's tribes. These are the indigenous methods used to educate its individuals in order for them to conform to society's rules.

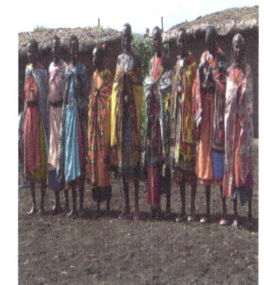

Detornosabroad.com

FGC is still practiced in some parts of Zimbabwe and is categorized as type 4, which involves the pulling of the labia majora until it is stretched to the extent that it protrudes between the woman's legs

Point to remember

Discuss any society rules, which may affect a woman accessing pregnancy care. This may be needed in order to tailor care that is culturally sensitive.

Diet

The staple food in Zimbabwe is sadza a maize-meal based dish which may be eaten with relish such as a vegetable or meat stew. Sadza is cooked slowly and is thicker than porridge. Common meats eaten are beef, chicken, pork and goat. Vegetables consist of green beans, butternut squash, cucumbers and avocados.

Pregnancy

Apart from marriage a woman's importance is enhanced by motherhood. This is the traditional norm of defining a woman's status. There are particular cultural taboos which are adhered to in the Shona tribes due to fear of infertility or harm to the child. Most religious or traditional practices relating to pregnancy and childbirth are followed to allow a successful pregnancy and childbirth. In Shona cosmology a woman's birth canal represents a temple for creation and signifies fertility and growth of the clan. Childlessness is an unnatural condition. Remedies for childlessness include the use of herbs and prayers.

Antenatal

When the pregnancy is in the first trimester this is felt to be the time that the woman is more at risk of witchcraft. Indigenous religions or even Christianity may be used as a mean of protecting the developing child. This may be done by use of prayers and using holy water.

Due to this fear of witchcraft only close family members are informed of the pregnancy. It is this point that may prevent a woman from attending for pregnancy care too early. Women may drink herbal remedies to prepare and relax the birth canal. Substances such as herbal pastes and soap are used as lubrication to stretch and massage the vagina, which is believed to ease the delivery of the baby. Traditionally, if the woman is having her first child she will stay with her parents for the last trimester of pregnancy and up to three months postnatally.

Point to remember

If may be important to question the woman about any practices regarding the stretching of the birth canal and provide advice particularly around issues such as risk of infection.

Labour

The Shona belief about pain is that it is to be tolerated; women are not expected to cry out, but to be silent and strong. Hence, because of this analgesia may not be accepted by some women. Enemas may be used to cleanse the bowel for labour. Some men still persist in not being present during the birth. It is believed that seeing the wife give birth may affect his sexual appetite.

Postnatal

The baby

The baby must be bathed straight after delivery because there is a belief that the child is dirty. The newborn baby must be kept in doors for two to three months to avoid risk of harm to the baby. Only in emergencies can the baby be taken outside. The cord once it has separated may be kept and sent home to elders for prayer and burial, this is to protect the baby.

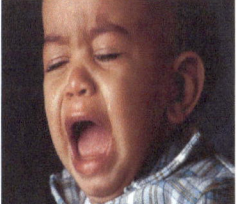

phillisremastered.wordpress.com

The mother

Breastfeeding is an accepted practice, but is advised to be performed only after the woman has washed. This is because the body is believed to be dirty after birth. Some woman may just use a cloth to wipe their breast prior to breastfeeding. The mother may tie her abdomen post-delivery to keep the stomach flat and aid evolution.

Bibliography

Chigidi Lungisani, W. 2009 Shona Taboos: The language of manufacturing fears for sustainable development, Journal of Pan African Studies, vol.3, no.1 pp. 174-187.

Mathole, T. Lindmark, G 2004 A Qualitative study of Women's Perspective of Antenatal Care in a Rural Area of Zimbabwe, Midwifery, vol. 20, no.2, pp. 122-132.

Meekers, D. 1993 The noble custom of roora: the marriage of the Shona of Zimbabwe, Ethnology, vol.32, pp.35-54.

Mungwini, P. 2008 Shona Womanhood: Rethinking Social Identities in the face of HIV in Zimbabwe, Journal of Pan African Studies, vol.2, no.4, pp.203-214.

Section five

CENTRAL AFRICAN CULTURE

5.1 CAMEROON

Cameroon is located in central Africa and is bordered by Nigeria to the west, the Central Republic of Africa and Chad to the east. Cameroon is a name given by the Portuguese to describe the Wouri river 'Rio dos Camroroes'. The name means river of prawns after the species of crayfish found there. The population of Cameroon is approximately 16 million. There are over 200 ethnic groups in Cameroon, which are divided into five large ethnic groups. The western highlanders are the Bamileke and Bamoun people, the central rain foresters are the Douala and the southern rain foresters, are the Beti, Bui and Fang people. In the northern and central regions are the Islamic people of Cameroon.

Languages

The main languages spoken are English, French and native tongue. There are over 250 local languages. English or French are spoken in school depending on the region. A majority of Cameroonian's are multilingual, a majority of people also speak French and their native tongue.

Religion

The main religion is Christianity (53%). Indigenous religious is practiced by approximately 25% of the population and 22% of Cameroonians practice Islam.

Society

Cameroon is a patrilineal society, where men acquire a higher status than woman. In social meetings a handshake is required with interest in the person and their families well being. Respect is always given to elders. Women have strict tribal roles and failure to comply is felt to cause bewitchment, illness or even death.

Female genital cutting is not widely practiced in Cameroon and it is becoming eradicated with increase in knowledge. Marriage in Cameroon is primarily for the purpose of rearing children.

Pregnancy

Pregnancy and childbirth are considered an illness in Cameroonian culture because of the high risk they pose to the mother. Practices are undertaken to ensure the well being of the fetus. Sperm is considered scared and is called white blood and is said to have benefits to the unborn fetus. Steps are taken to improve conception by not allowing mixing of menses blood and the sperm. Conception as well as being a physical event is seen as a blessing from divine powers. Herbs are also used to protect the pregnancy, this may be a concoction made into an enema.

Diet

The Cameroonian diet consists of cooked cereal or root staples eaten with a sauce or stew. The common staples are cassava, cocoyam and plantain. The sauce and stews are usually made from palm oil or ground peanuts to

Now-here-this.timeout.com

which dried fish or meat is added. Common vegetables eaten are greens, okra, squashes, hot peppers, onions, ginger and tomatoes. Bananas, mangoes, papayas, oranges and avocados are popular snacks and are not considered part of a meal.

Foods that woman may avoid during pregnancy to maintain maternal well being

Food	Reason
Birds	Prevents development of breasts
Pig	Child may be born to big
Duck	Child maybe born with rickets
Pineapple/banana	Child may be born covered with scabs, sores, scratches or oedema
Taro	Child may be born covered in dirt, prevents closing of fontanelle
Beans	Cause problem with child's spleen
Sugarcane	Reduces quality of milk

Any food that causes sickness in the mother is thought to be a rejection from the fetus. Some tribes encourage pregnant women to eat vegetable soup in order to increase milk supply at birth. Large quantities of gourd leaves, okra and cassava are also consumed during pregnancy. Women also eat Kaolin (white clay), which is said to protect the fetus and strengthen its bones.

Point to remember

Inform the woman of common pregnancy ailments and causes of these so that she does not avoid foods that have nutritional value because of cultural assumptions

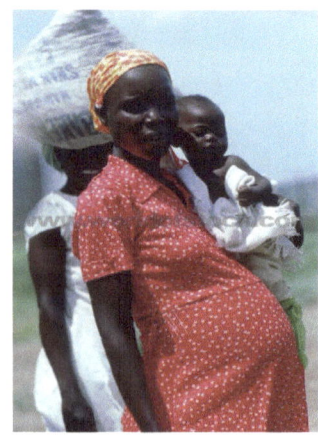

Srxaworldonhealth.com

Antenatal

Pregnancy is normally kept secret for the first trimester from others apart from close relatives; in the some tribes even the husband is not informed. This is to prevent harm from malevolent spirits. In one tribe after menses has ceased during pregnancy even sexual intercourse is avoided. Sexual intercourse is also avoided at seven to eight months in order to avoid soiling the fetus and causing hyperthermia at birth.

Cameroonians believe that a child sees and hears all that the mother encounters. The child is supposed to resemble what is sees, hence a pregnant woman allows a person with delicate features to pass or sleep behind her. On the other hand a pregnant woman will avoid a person who has unattractive features. The fetus is believed to control the mother's physical needs, so nausea, diarrhoea, cramp or flatulence in the mother is a sign that the fetus is refusing food from the mother. If the mother is hungry then this signifies that the fetus wants more food and frequency of urine in the mother is interpreted as a sign that the baby needs to urinate.

A pregnant woman should avoid conflict during her pregnancy, avoid touching other people's property, offending a child or harming a domestic animal this is to avoid a difficult labour or miscarriage. Any association with the dead is considered harmful to pregnancy, including entering the house of the deceased or attending the funeral. If a woman's baby becomes overdue a child it is considered to be sleeping and is not ready for an external environment, or start of labour has been delayed by the will of transcendental powers. The length of gestation is believed to be dependent on the sex of the child or whether the woman is carrying twins. A woman carries a baby for less than nine months for a girl and more than nine months for a boy according to Cameroonian beliefs.

Point to remember

Discuss with the women the importance of induction of labour if the baby is overdue. Having this conversation may dispel any fears on the woman's part.

Labour

Childbirth is a woman's matter and men may not attend. The woman is give plenty of fluids to drink, this may consist of herbs with oxytocic properties. The position adopted is normally a semi seated or all fours position. Prayers are said which are thought to help with easing the woman's pain.

Postnatal

The baby

The placenta, umbilical cord and mother's breast are believed to be connected. Hence, the placenta will be hidden secretly so that no spells can be used against the mother or baby. Bandaging of the cord is practised by mothers and the use of traditional substances on the umbilicus. Another common practice is the use of eye drops for two to seven days. Breastfeeding is a common practice, although the use of water is common. This is due to pressure from elders and families as giving water is a traditional practice.

Point to remember

It is important to discuss with the mother the use of any other fluids used to supplement breastfeed and be aware of family influences.

The mother

After birth the mother may be massaged and washed with hot water and given herbal drinks and soups to increase her strength and to remove any blood from the womb which is believed to cause pain and flatulence. As sperm is considered scared any interference with it is considered taboo, so any method of contraception or withdrawal methods are taboo.

Bibliography

Beninguisse, G. De Brouwere, V. 2004 Tradition and Modernity in Cameroon: The Confrontation between Social Demand and Biomedical Logics of Health Service, African Journal Reproductive Health, vol. 8, no.3, pp.152-175.

Kakute, P.N. Ngum, J. Mitchell, P. Kroll, K.A. Forgwei, G W. Ngwang, L K. Meyer, D J. 2013 Cultural barriers to exclusive breastfeeding by mothers in a rural area of Cameroon, Africa, Journal of Midwifery Women's Health, vol.50, no.4, pp.324-8.

Weinger, S. 2007 Cameroonian Women's Perception of their Health Needs, Nordic Journal of African Studies, vol. 16, no.1, pp.47-63.